Eat Well

Live

Vibrantly

Your Guide to Weight Loss and

Health-Boosting Foods

KARRY WILSON

Table of Contents

INTRODUCTION

In a world where fast-paced lives often dictate our choices, the significance of what we put on our plates cannot be overstated. Welcome to "Eat Well, Live Vibrantly: Your Guide to Weight Loss and Health-Boosting Foods," a journey into the heart of nutrition's transformative power. In these pages, we embark on a quest to redefine not just our diets but our very lives.

Imagine a life where each meal is a step towards a healthier, happier you. It's not a fantasy; it's a tangible reality waiting to be embraced. The foods we consume have the remarkable ability to shape our bodies and minds, to heal and rejuvenate, to ignite our energy and resilience. This isn't just about shedding pounds; it's about rediscovering your vitality, your zest for life.

Here, we'll unlock the secrets of 36 potent foods, carefully curated to help you shed excess weight and, more importantly, boost your overall well-being. These foods aren't just ingredients; they are your allies on a journey towards a more vibrant, healthier you.

So, whether you're starting your wellness journey or seeking to refine your approach, "Eat Well, Live Vibrantly" is your compass. It's a guide that transcends fad diets and quick fixes, leading you towards a sustainable, fulfilling, and delicious way of life. Let's embark on this adventure together, discovering the magic that happens when you choose to nourish your body and soul with intention.

CHAPTER 1

The Science of Fat Loss

In today's world, where body image and health are paramount, it's crucial to understand that being overweight doesn't define your worth. It's simply a state of being. However, shedding those extra pounds can lead to increased self-esteem, better health, and a sense of pride.

Once you've embarked on your weight loss journey, maintaining your newfound vitality becomes the next chapter.

In the following pages, we'll delve into a revolutionary approach to weight loss – one that allows you to shed 10 pounds a month, a safe and sustainable loss of approximately two to two-and-a-half pounds per week.

The best part? You'll do it without feeling deprived or drained; instead, you'll feel satisfied and energized like never before.

The journey to success starts with understanding that most weight gain results from poor dietary choices. Transforming these habits is the foundation of your long-term triumph. Knowledge, coupled with the right nutrition, will be your guiding light.

In ancient times, our ancestors lived as hunter-gatherers, blissfully unaware of food preservation. Their existence revolved around hunting and gathering, and when they found food, they consumed it swiftly. Instead of stocking pantries, they stored energy within their bodies in the form of fat, ready to burn during lean times.

Each year, it was essential for them to accumulate a layer of fat during abundant seasons to ensure survival during harsh winters. This strategy was particularly crucial for women who bore and nurtured the tribe's future generation, requiring extra energy.

While our lifestyles have evolved beyond caves, this fundamental fat storage mechanism remains ingrained in our biology.

We are all born with a specific number of fat cells, a genetic legacy. Having more fat cells can be an ancestral advantage, as larger individuals had higher survival odds.

You cannot eliminate fat cells, but you can shrink them. When you lose weight, you're essentially burning the stored fat within these cells. Visualize them as balloons; weight loss is akin to releasing the air from these balloons.

Effective weight management involves calorie restriction, consuming fewer calories than you expend. This process shrinks fat cells, leading to weight loss.

However, sustainable success hinges on more than just calorie counting. To achieve lasting results, you must alter your food choices to reduce fat intake while ensuring your body receives essential nutrients such as vitamins, minerals, trace elements, protein, fats, and carbohydrates.

Crash diets, while promising rapid weight loss, ultimately fail in the long term. Our bodies are hardwired to safeguard against starvation by slowing metabolism during food shortages. A crucial part of our brain called the hypothalamus establishes a "set point" for our comfortable weight, even if it exceeds healthy levels.

Drastically reducing food intake triggers the brain to believe the body is starving, prompting a metabolic slowdown, and weight loss plateaus. This leads to discomfort and increased hunger, ultimately derailing the diet.

To counteract this metabolic slowdown, you must modify your food's nutritional composition. Reducing total calories is fundamental, but equally crucial is decreasing the percentage of calories derived from fat. This prevents your body from entering starvation mode.

By replacing high-fat foods with nutrient-rich, low-calorie plant-based alternatives, you'll signal to your brain that it's receiving the necessary nutrition. This strategic shift allows you to eat more food, feel satisfied, and consume fewer calories and fats.

Plant-based foods digest slowly, promoting a prolonged feeling of fullness. They're rich in essential nutrients like vitamins, minerals, trace elements, carbohydrates, and protein, providing energy and supporting muscle growth. This transformation empowers your body to efficiently

burn stored fat, finally achieving the weight loss and health
you desire.

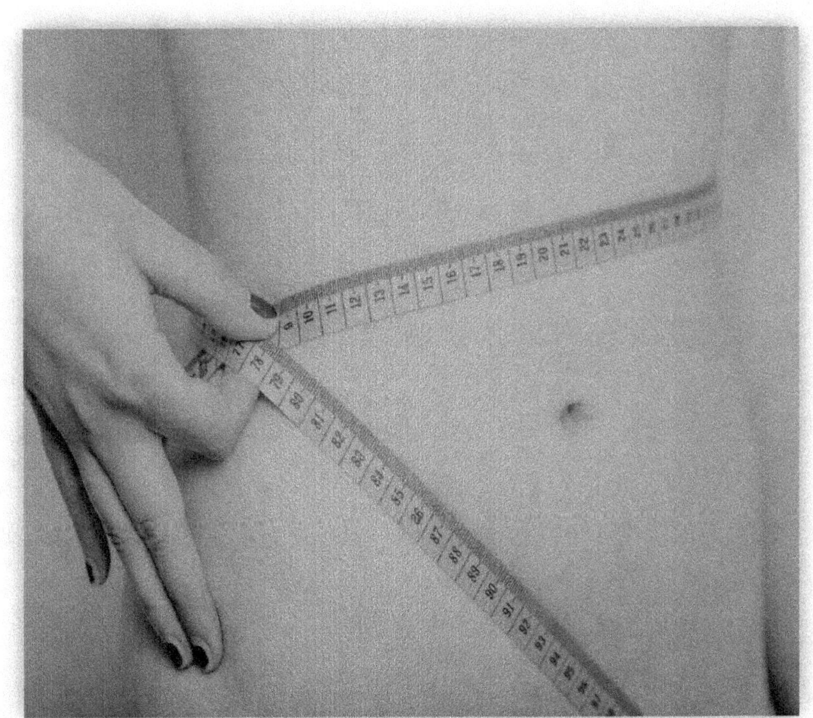

CHAPTER 2

The Fat-Burning Revolution

Welcome to a new era of fat loss, where we unveil a modern and effective approach to melting those unwanted pounds. The foods we introduce are not just calorie-free; they are superheroes in the world of nutrition, equipped with unique abilities to ignite your metabolism and help you achieve your weight loss goals. These powerhouse foods are not just about losing weight; they're about revolutionizing your entire relationship with food and health.

Apples: Nature's Doctor Away

Apples have long been hailed for their health benefits, and they're not just keeping doctors at bay. These fruits now also help you trim down. They gently elevate your blood glucose levels, providing a prolonged sense of satisfaction. Apples are also rich in soluble fiber, which prevents hunger pangs by stabilizing blood sugar levels. Furthermore, they offer a host of additional health perks, such as lowering cholesterol and blood pressure.

Whole Grain Bread: The Misunderstood Hero

It's time to dispel the myth that bread is the enemy. In reality, it's what you spread on it that matters. Whole grain bread, packed with fiber and complex carbohydrates, is your ally in weight loss. Studies show that it can even reduce appetite, making it a valuable addition to your diet.

Coffee: The Wake-Up Call to Your Metabolism

For coffee lovers, here's some good news. Moderate coffee consumption can kickstart your metabolism, thanks to its caffeine content. While too much caffeine can lead to anxiety and insomnia, a cup or two a day can boost your calorie burn by up to 10 percent. Opt for skim milk and consider skipping sugar to keep it a healthy choice.

Grapefruit: The Natural Fat Fighter

Grapefruit has earned its reputation as a diet-friendly fruit for good reason. It's a potent fat and cholesterol dissolver. Rich in pectin, vitamin C, and potassium, it supports heart health and weight loss. To balance its tartness, try a sprinkle of cinnamon instead of sugar.

Mustard: Spice Up Your Metabolism

Spicy mustard varieties, especially those found in Asian cuisine, can temporarily accelerate your metabolism, similar to caffeine. Natural and safe, mustard can boost your calorie burn by up to 25 percent for several hours, making it a valuable addition to your diet.

Peppers: The Fiery Metabolism Boosters

Chili peppers, known for their heat, share a metabolism-boosting trait with mustard. Even a small amount can create a diet-induced thermic effect, causing your body to burn extra calories. Beyond their fat-burning prowess, peppers are rich in vitamins and minerals while being low in calories.

Potatoes: The Surprising Weight Loss Allies

Contrary to popular belief, potatoes are not the villains they're made out to be. A single potato contains just 85 calories and is rich in fiber and potassium. When prepared wisely (sans butter, milk, or sour cream), they're a fantastic addition to your diet.

Rice: The Staple of Success

The Rice Diet, founded in the 1930s, has demonstrated exceptional weight loss and health benefits. A cup of cooked rice is remarkably low in calories, around 178, making it an ideal base for a weight-loss plan when paired with fruits and vegetables.

Soups: A Bowl of Weight Loss

Old-fashioned homemade soups can play a crucial role in weight loss. Research suggests that having soup before meals can lead to more significant weight loss and sustained results. Opt for broth-based soups, as cream soups can be calorie-dense.

Spinach: Popeye's Secret Weapon

Popeye was onto something with his spinach obsession. This leafy green lowers cholesterol, fires up your metabolism, and aids in burning fat. Rich in vitamins and iron, it's a nutritional powerhouse.

Tofu: The Versatile Protein

Tofu, or soybean curd, is a blank canvas for flavors. It's low in calories and saturated fat, a source of calcium and iron, and an excellent protein provider. It revs up your metabolism and can even lower cholesterol.

These foods represent the modern era of fat loss. They're not just about shedding pounds but revolutionizing the way we view nutrition and health. Incorporate them wisely into your diet, and witness the transformation of your body and well-being.

CHAPTER 3

The Powerhouse Foods Revolution

In a world filled with tantalizing culinary options, we understand that a successful weight loss journey requires more than just a few staple foods. So, we present a new lineup of nutritional heavyweights to accompany the fantastic foods introduced in our previous section.

These newcomers offer diverse tastes and textures to your meals while supplying an array of essential vitamins, minerals, proteins, and other crucial nutrients. And the best part? They're brimming with fiber, low in fat, and sodium-conscious.

Barley: The Ancient Grain Reimagined

Barley, often overshadowed by rice and potatocs, is reclaiming its place as a nutritional powerhouse. With 170 calories per cooked cup, it boasts commendable levels of protein and fiber while keeping fat content low.

Notably, Roman gladiators relied on barley for strength. Research at the University of Wisconsin demonstrates barley's potential to lower cholesterol by up to 15 percent and its potent anti-cancer properties.

Barley can also aid digestion, making it a weight loss-friendly grain. Use it as a rice substitute, incorporate it into salads, pilafs, and soups, or combine it with rice for an exciting twist.

Beans: The Plant Protein Heroes

Beans, including peas, chickpeas, and more, reign supreme as plant-based protein sources. Most common beans offer about 215 calories per cooked cup, making them the leanest protein choice. They're rich in potassium and remarkably low in sodium.

To unlock their full protein potential, pair beans with whole grains like rice, barley, or corn. This combination provides a complete protein source that rivals meat in quality but with a fraction of the fat.

Regular bean consumption has even been linked to reduced cholesterol levels.

Berries: Nature's Sweet Satisfaction

Berries are the ultimate weight loss treat, balancing natural fructose sugar with substantial fiber to keep calorie absorption in check. British research highlights the benefits of insoluble fiber in reducing calorie absorption from foods, aiding in weight loss without compromising nutrition.

Berries also contribute to potassium intake, helping regulate blood pressure. Blackberries, blueberries, raspberries, and strawberries all come in under 100 calories per cup, providing a delightful array of choices.

Broccoli: America's Green Gem

With a mere 44 calories per cooked cup, broccoli is America's beloved vegetable, prized for its nutritional prowess. It boasts zero fat, high fiber content, cancer-fighting indoles, a wealth of carotene, an astounding 21 times the recommended daily intake of vitamin C, and a generous dose of calcium.

Look for bright green, non-yellowing florets and firm stems when purchasing.

Buckwheat: The Unsung Grain

Buckwheat, whether in pancakes, bread, cereal, or kasha, offers 155 calories per cooked cup. Research from the All India Institute of Medical Sciences underscores its blood sugar-regulating properties, resistance to diabetes, and cholesterol-lowering effects. Preparing buckwheat is as straightforward as rice or barley: bring two to three cups of water to a boil, add the grain, cover, reduce heat, and simmer for 20 minutes or until the water is absorbed.

Cabbage: The Eastern European Gem

Cabbage, a staple in Eastern European cuisine, is a dietary wonder at a mere 33 calories per cooked cup. Whether eaten raw, cooked, as sauerkraut, or coleslaw, cabbage offers protection against colon cancer and potentially enhances longevity. It's an excellent choice for those looking to shed pounds without feeling deprived.

Carrots: Bugs Bunny's Favorite for a Reason

Carrots, one of nature's perfect snacks, are both flavorful and nutritious, containing around 55 calories per medium-sized carrot. Their vibrant orange hue hints at their beta carotene content, a potent cancer-preventing nutrient. Incorporate them into various dishes, from pasta to stir-fries, to add a delightful natural sweetness.

Chicken: Lean Protein Powerhouse

Chicken provides a lean source of protein, with white meat offering 245 calories per four-ounce serving and dark meat, 285. Rich in protein, iron, niacin, and zinc, chicken is a versatile choice for health-conscious individuals. Opt for skinless chicken to keep it lean while retaining moisture during cooking.

Corn: The Underrated Grain

Corn, often overlooked as a grain, packs a nutritional punch at 178 calories per cup of cooked kernels. It supplies ample iron, zinc, and potassium while providing high-quality protein.

The Tarahumara Indians of Mexico, whose diet revolves around corn and beans, demonstrate low rates of high cholesterol and heart disease. Corn is a versatile ingredient, whether in its whole form or incorporated into various dishes.

Cottage Cheese: The Versatile Dairy Delight

Low-fat (2%) cottage cheese, with 205 calories per cup, is a dairy superstar. Packed with calcium and riboflavin, it serves as an ideal canvas for flavor experimentation. Season it with herbs or pair it with fruits for a satisfying, low-calorie treat. Cottage cheese can also replace higher-fat ingredients in recipes, making it a smart choice for health-conscious cooks.

Figs: Fiber-Rich Delights

Figs, rich in fiber and low in calories (37 per medium raw fig), contribute to a sense of fullness and prevent overeating. They are a perfect addition to a fruit and cheese platter or a sweet pastry filling. These versatile fruits elevate both taste and nutrition in various dishes.

Fish: The Heart-Healthy Option

Fish, renowned for its heart health benefits, delivers an array of options. Deep-sea fish, from abalone to herring, range from 90 to 236 calories per four-ounce serving. Fish oils thin the blood, lower blood pressure, and reduce cholesterol, all contributing to heart health. Fish also aids in conditions like rheumatoid arthritis.

Greens: Leafy Marvels

Collard, chicory, beet, kale, mustard, Swiss chard, and turnip greens are dietary superheroes, offering less than 50 calories per cooked cup. These greens are fiber-rich, high in vitamins A and C, and completely fat-free. Use them interchangeably with spinach in salads, soups, casseroles, and any spinach-based dish.

Kiwi: The Exotic Vitamin C Bomb

Kiwi, a fruit from New Zealand, contains a mere 46 calories per fruit and is praised for its high vitamin C content and potassium. Its versatility in cooking or as a snack makes it an excellent addition to a weight loss regimen.

Leeks: Flavorful and Low-Calorie

Leeks, cousins of scallions, contribute a mere 32 calories per cooked cup and offer rich flavor. Poach, broil, marinate, or incorporate them into soups and dishes to savor their taste and health benefits.

Lettuce: More than Just Greens

Lettuce, often underestimated, is a calorie-saving superstar at just 10 calories per cup of raw romaine. Beyond iceberg lettuce, explore Boston, bibb, cos, watercress, arugula, radicchio, dandelion greens, purslane, and parsley to elevate your salads.

Melons: Sweetness in a Low-Calorie Package

Cantaloupe, casaba, honeydew, and watermelon offer sweetness and nutrition with calorie counts ranging from 44 to 62 per cup. These high-fiber fruits also pack a punch of vitamins A and C, along with ample potassium.

Oats: The Satiety Grain

Oats, with only 110 calories per cup, are a satiating breakfast option. Studies show that incorporating oats into your diet can promote weight loss. However, remember that a balanced diet is essential for overall health.

Onions: Flavorful and Nutritious

Onions, renowned for their flavor, come in at 60 calories per cup of chopped raw onions. They offer cholesterol control, blood-thinning properties, and potential allergy relief. Onions are versatile in cooking and pair well with various ingredients.

Pasta: The Italian Staple

Pasta, with 155 calories per cooked cup (without heavy sauces), is a perfect base for your meals. Whole wheat pasta is an even healthier option. It's rich in essential minerals and provides a solid foundation for a balanced diet.

Sweet Potatoes: Nutrient-Rich Delights

Sweet potatoes, at approximately 103 calories each, are a satiating choice. Their creamy orange flesh is a vitamin A powerhouse. Incorporate them into various dishes, from baking to soups, and savor their natural sweetness.

Tomatoes: The Garden's Treasures

A medium tomato boasts only about 25 calories, making it a low-fat, low-sodium, and fiber-rich option. Regular tomato consumption is associated with lower cancer rates, especially when combined with strawberries. Explore canned tomato varieties to enhance sauces, casseroles, and soups.

Turkey: The Lean Poultry Marvel

Turkey, whether white or dark meat, offers lean protein with 177 to 211 calories per four-ounce serving. Ground turkey is a versatile alternative to ground beef, significantly lowering calorie and fat intake.

Yogurt: The Dairy Delight

Non-fat plain yogurt contains 120 calories per cup, while low-fat has 144. Yogurt is a protein powerhouse, rich in calcium, zinc, and riboflavin. It's versatile in both sweet and savory dishes, making it a valuable addition to your diet.

These nutritional powerhouses redefine weight loss by combining taste and health in every bite. Experiment, create, and enjoy a diverse and satisfying menu that keeps you on track toward your weight loss goals.

CHAPTER 4

Seeds of Wellness: Nuts and Seeds

Welcome to the world of nuts and seeds, where small packages deliver mighty nutrition. In this chapter, we'll explore how these tiny powerhouses can be your secret weapons on the journey to wellness and weight loss. Nuts and seeds are not only delicious but also packed with essential nutrients that support your overall health.

The Nutritional Bounty of Nuts

Nuts, despite their small size, are loaded with nutrients that can benefit your body in numerous ways. They are rich in healthy fats, including monounsaturated and polyunsaturated fats, which are known to support heart health. These fats can help reduce bad cholesterol levels, lowering the risk of heart disease.

Additionally, nuts are excellent sources of plant-based protein, making them a valuable addition to vegetarian and vegan diets. Protein helps with satiety, keeping those hunger pangs at bay. When you feel fuller for longer, you're less likely to indulge in unhealthy snacking.

Fiber is another nutritional gem found in nuts. It aids in digestion and can contribute to a feeling of fullness. Moreover, nuts provide an array of essential vitamins and minerals, including vitamin E, magnesium, and potassium.

The Benefits of Seeds

Seeds, like nuts, are nutritional powerhouses. They come in various forms, from chia and flax seeds to sunflower and pumpkin seeds. Each type offers unique health benefits.

For instance, chia seeds are renowned for their high fiber content. When mixed with liquid, they form a gel-like consistency that can help control appetite and support healthy digestion. Flax seeds are a fantastic source of omega-3 fatty acids, which are essential for heart health and may aid in weight loss.

Sunflower and pumpkin seeds are rich in vitamins and minerals like vitamin E, folate, and selenium. These nutrients play vital roles in maintaining overall health, from supporting a strong immune system to promoting healthy skin.

Incorporating Nuts and Seeds into Your Diet

Now that we've uncovered the nutritional treasures within nuts and seeds, let's explore how to make them a delicious part of your daily diet:

Snacking Smart: Instead of reaching for chips or cookies, opt for a handful of mixed nuts or seeds. Create your own trail mix by combining your favorites with dried fruits for a satisfying, nutrient-rich snack.

Morning Boost: Sprinkle chia or flax seeds on your morning cereal, yogurt, or oatmeal. This quick addition not only enhances the taste but also increases the fiber content to keep you full until your next meal.

Salads with Crunch: Toss some seeds or chopped nuts onto your salads. They add a delightful crunch and boost the nutritional value of your greens.

Smooth Operator: Blend nuts into your morning smoothie. They'll not only add creaminess but also a dose of healthy fats and protein.

Nutty Spreads: Swap out your regular peanut butter for almond, cashew, or sunflower seed butter. Spread it on whole-grain bread or use it as a dip for fresh fruit and vegetables.

Cooking with Seeds: Experiment with seeds as an ingredient in recipes. Try incorporating sunflower seeds into your stir-fry or adding toasted sesame seeds to your favorite dishes for a burst of flavor and nutrition.

Baking Delights: Use ground nuts or seeds as a flour substitute in baking. This can make your baked goods more nutrient-dense while adding a delightful nutty flavor.

Portion Control is Key

While nuts and seeds offer an array of health benefits, it's essential to consume them in moderation. They are calorie-dense, meaning that even a small amount can contribute a significant number of calories to your diet. To avoid overindulging, pre-portion your snacks or meals that include nuts and seeds.

Nuts and seeds are indeed seeds of wellness. They provide a wealth of nutrients, healthy fats, and protein, making them an excellent choice for those on a weight loss journey or anyone striving to improve their overall health. By incorporating these small but mighty foods into your diet, you'll be on your way to vibrant living and a healthier, happier you.

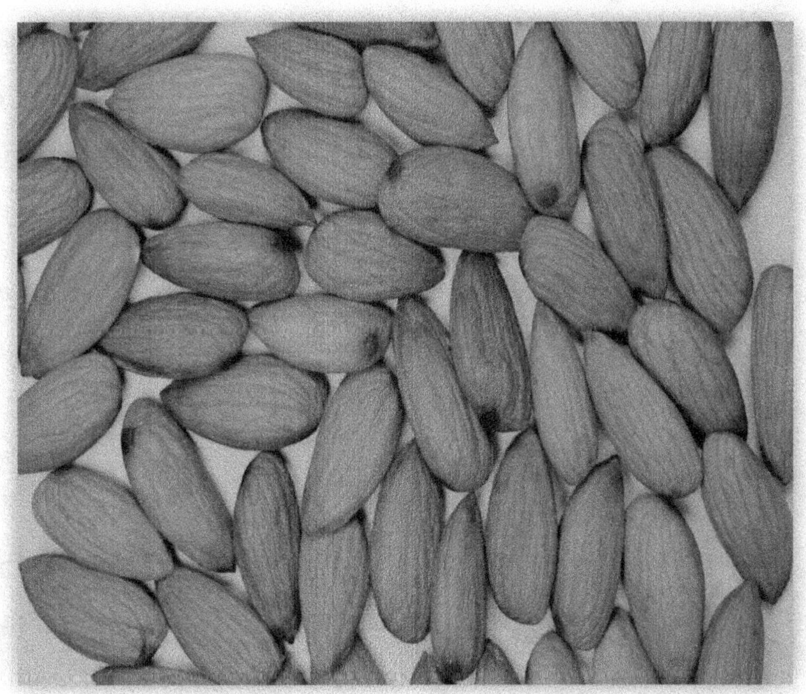

CHAPTER 5

Nature's Liquid Gold: Herbal Teas and Infusions

In this chapter, we delve into the world of herbal teas and infusions, where age-old wisdom meets modern wellness. These beverages, often referred to as "nature's liquid gold," have been cherished for centuries for their various health benefits.

Let's explore how incorporating herbal teas and infusions into your daily routine can be a delightful and nutritious way to support your well-being.

The Essence of Herbal Teas and Infusions

Herbal teas and infusions are made by steeping dried herbs, flowers, fruits, or other plant materials in hot water. Unlike traditional teas such as green, black, or oolong tea, which are derived from the Camellia sinensis plant, herbal teas are caffeine-free, making them a gentle and soothing choice any time of the day or night.

A Sip of Wellness

The beauty of herbal teas lies not only in their delightful flavors but also in their potential health-promoting properties. Depending on the herbs used, these infusions can aid in digestion, relaxation, immunity boosting, and more. Here are some popular herbal teas and their benefits:

Chamomile Tea: Chamomile, known for its calming and soothing effects, can help alleviate stress and promote better sleep. It may also aid digestion and relieve stomach discomfort.

Peppermint Tea: Peppermint tea is a natural remedy for indigestion, bloating, and nausea. It's also invigorating and can help increase alertness.

Ginger Tea: Ginger is renowned for its anti-inflammatory properties and can assist with nausea relief, especially during pregnancy or motion sickness. It may also help soothe sore throats and reduce muscle pain.

Lavender Tea: Lavender tea is excellent for relaxation and stress reduction. A cup before bedtime can help induce a peaceful night's sleep.

Echinacea Tea: Often used as a natural remedy for the common cold, echinacea tea can boost your immune system and reduce the severity and duration of cold symptoms.

Hibiscus Tea: Packed with antioxidants, hibiscus tea can help lower blood pressure, improve liver health, and support weight management.

Brewing the Perfect Cup

Brewing herbal teas and infusions is a simple and enjoyable process. Here's a basic guide to get you started:

Choose Quality Ingredients: Select high-quality dried herbs or herbal tea blends from reputable sources. Organic options are often preferred to ensure purity.

Boil Fresh Water: Heat fresh, cold water to a rolling boil. Avoid using water that has been sitting for an extended period, as it may have a flat taste.

Measure and Steep: Use about one teaspoon of dried herbs or a tea bag per 8-ounce cup. Place the herbs in a teapot or cup, and pour the hot water over them. Cover and let steep for the recommended time (usually 5-10 minutes, but it can vary depending on the type of herb).

Sweeten and Flavor (Optional): Add honey, lemon, or your preferred sweetener and flavorings to taste. Some herbal teas are delightful on their own, while others benefit from a touch of sweetness

Enjoy Mindfully: Sip slowly, savoring each sip. Herbal teas are meant to be a calming and pleasurable experience, so take your time.

Incorporating Herbal Teas into Your Daily Routine

Making herbal teas and infusions a regular part of your daily routine is a simple yet effective way to support your overall well-being. Here are some tips for incorporating them into your life:

Morning Wake-Up: Replace your usual morning coffee with an invigorating herbal tea like peppermint or ginger for a caffeine-free energy boost.

Afternoon Calm: Combat afternoon stress or fatigue with a cup of chamomile or lavender tea to help you relax and recenter.

Pre-Meal Ritual: Enjoy a cup of hibiscus tea before meals to aid digestion and potentially support weight management.

Bedtime Bliss: Create a soothing bedtime routine by sipping on calming herbal teas like chamomile or valerian root to enhance sleep quality.

Immunity Boost: During cold and flu season, incorporate echinacea tea into your routine to strengthen your immune system.

Hydration Helper: Herbal teas can count toward your daily hydration needs, so keep a variety on hand to enjoy throughout the day.

Liquid Gold for Well-Being

Herbal teas and infusions are gifts from nature, offering a myriad of flavors and potential health benefits. Whether you're seeking relaxation, better sleep, digestion support, or immune-boosting properties, there's an herbal tea to suit your needs. By embracing these natural elixirs, you're not only nurturing your body but also engaging in a delightful and healthful daily ritual that can enhance your overall quality of life. Cheers to sipping your way to wellness with nature's liquid gold!

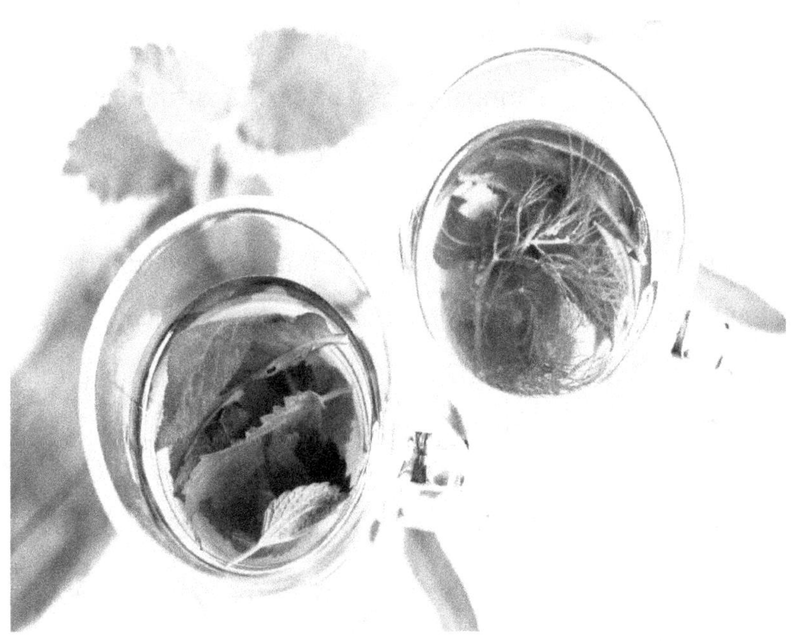

CHAPTER 6

Spice Up Your Life: The Magic of Herbs and Spices

In this chapter, we embark on a flavorful journey into the captivating world of herbs and spices. These tiny powerhouses of taste have not only transformed bland dishes into culinary masterpieces but also wield an array of health benefits. Let's explore how you can spice up your life with herbs and spices, turning every meal into a mouthwatering and health-boosting experience.

Herbs vs. Spices: Unveiling the Difference

Before we dive into the magic of herbs and spices, it's essential to understand the distinction between the two:

Herbs: Herbs are the leafy, green parts of plants used for flavoring. These typically come from the leaves of various plants and are often used fresh or dried. Examples include basil, parsley, mint, and cilantro.

Spices: Spices, on the other hand, are derived from the seeds, bark, roots, or fruits of plants and are typically dried. These are known for their potent flavors and aromas. Examples include cinnamon, cumin, paprika, and ginger.

Both herbs and spices offer unique tastes and aromas that can elevate your dishes, but they also bring a host of health benefits to the table.

The Health Benefits of Herbs and Spices

Herbs and spices are not just culinary delights; they are also nature's pharmacy. Here are some remarkable health benefits associated with these flavor-packed ingredients:

Antioxidant Powerhouses: Many herbs and spices, such as turmeric, oregano, and cinnamon, are rich in antioxidants. These compounds help combat oxidative stress in the body, reducing the risk of chronic diseases like cancer and heart disease.

Anti-Inflammatory Allies: Chronic inflammation is a root cause of various health issues. Spices like ginger and garlic, along with herbs like rosemary and thyme, possess anti-inflammatory properties that can help reduce inflammation and associated ailments.

Digestive Aids: Herbs like peppermint and fennel, as well as spices like cumin and coriander, have been used for centuries to aid digestion, alleviate bloating, and soothe an upset stomach.

Blood Sugar Control: Some spices, including cinnamon and fenugreek, have shown promise in helping regulate blood sugar levels, making them valuable for individuals with diabetes or those looking to manage their weight.

Heart Health: Spices like cayenne pepper and herbs like basil can support heart health by improving circulation and reducing blood pressure.

Enhanced Immunity: Garlic, known for its immune-boosting properties, is a staple in many cuisines. It can help strengthen your body's defense against infections.

Brain Health: Turmeric, thanks to its active compound curcumin, has been linked to improved cognitive function and a reduced risk of neurodegenerative diseases like Alzheimer's.

Harnessing the Magic of Herbs and Spices

Incorporating herbs and spices into your daily diet doesn't have to be complicated. Here are some tips to help you harness their magic:

Experiment Liberally: Don't be afraid to experiment with various herbs and spices. Each has a unique flavor profile that can transform your dishes. Start with small amounts and adjust to your taste.

Fresh vs. Dried: While fresh herbs offer vibrant flavors, dried herbs and spices have a longer shelf life. Use fresh herbs in salads and as garnishes and dried herbs and spices for cooking.

Pairing Perfection: Certain herbs and spices pair exceptionally well with specific foods. For example, rosemary complements roasted meats, while cinnamon enhances baked goods and oatmeal.

Balance is Key: Achieve a harmonious flavor balance by combining different herbs and spices. For instance, a pinch of cinnamon and nutmeg can elevate your morning coffee or oatmeal.

Homemade Spice Blends: Create your spice blends to have full control over flavors and avoid preservatives found in store-bought versions. Experiment with combinations like Italian seasoning or curry powder.

Mindful Storage: Store dried herbs and spices in airtight containers away from heat and light to preserve their potency.

A Dash of Flavor, A Pinch of Health

Herbs and spices are not only culinary delights but also powerful tools for enhancing your health. By incorporating a variety of these flavor-packed ingredients into your meals, you can elevate your dishes to new heights and reap the benefits of their remarkable health-boosting properties. So go ahead, spice up your life, and savor the magic of herbs and spices with every bite. Your taste buds and your well-being will thank you.

CHAPTER 7

Lean and Green: Plant-Based Proteins

In this chapter, we delve into the exciting world of plant-based proteins. As more people embrace the benefits of a plant-forward diet, the demand for tasty, nutritious, and sustainable protein sources has skyrocketed.

Let's explore the diverse and delicious world of plant-based proteins and discover how they can not only meet but exceed your nutritional needs.

The Rise of Plant-Based Proteins

Plant-based proteins have rapidly gained popularity for several compelling reasons:

Health Benefits: Plant-based diets have been linked to reduced risk factors for chronic diseases, including heart disease, diabetes, and certain cancers.

They are typically low in saturated fats and high in fiber, vitamins, minerals, and antioxidants.

Sustainability: Producing plant-based proteins generally requires fewer natural resources like land and water compared to raising livestock. This makes plant-based diets more environmentally friendly and sustainable.

Ethical Considerations: Concerns about animal welfare have prompted many individuals to explore plant-based protein sources as a compassionate alternative to traditional meat.

Variety and Flavor: The world of plant-based proteins is incredibly diverse, offering a wide range of flavors, textures, and culinary possibilities. From beans and lentils to tofu and tempeh, there's something for everyone.

Diverse Plant-Based Protein Sources

Let's take a closer look at some popular and versatile plant-based protein sources:

Legumes: Beans, lentils, and chickpeas are protein powerhouses.

They are rich in fiber, vitamins, and minerals while being low in fat. Whether you're making a hearty chili, a flavorful curry, or a zesty salad, legumes are a go-to choice.

Tofu: Tofu, made from soybeans, is an incredibly versatile protein source. It takes on the flavors of the ingredients it's cooked with, making it ideal for stir-fries, scrambles, and marinated dishes.

Tempeh: Another soy-based product, tempeh, is a fermented food that's dense in protein and has a nutty flavor. It's excellent for grilling, sautéing, or crumbling into tacos and salads.

Nuts: Almonds, peanuts, and cashews are not only delicious snacks but also great sources of plant-based protein. Nut butter and nut milk are easy ways to incorporate them into your diet.

Seeds: Chia seeds, flaxseeds, and hemp seeds are packed with protein, healthy fats, and fiber. Sprinkle them on yogurt, add them to smoothies, or use them as egg substitutes in baking.

Whole Grains: Quinoa, farro, and bulgur are examples of whole grains that contain significant amounts of protein. They can serve as a base for salads, side dishes, or breakfast bowls.

Vegetables: Certain vegetables like broccoli, spinach, and Brussels sprouts offer surprising amounts of protein. While they may not be as protein-rich as legumes or tofu, they contribute to your overall intake.

Balancing Your Plant-Based Diet

To ensure you're getting a balanced diet with all the essential nutrients, keep these tips in mind:

Combine Protein Sources: By mixing different plant-based proteins, you can create complete protein sources that contain all the essential amino acids your body needs.

Eat a Rainbow: Consume a variety of fruits and vegetables to maximize your intake of vitamins, minerals, and antioxidants.

Don't Forget Healthy Fats: Include sources of healthy fats like avocados, olive oil, and nuts in your meals for satiety and overall health.

Supplement Wisely: Consider supplements like vitamin B12 and iron if your plant-based diet may be deficient in these nutrients.

Experiment and Enjoy: Plant-based cooking is an adventure. Explore new recipes, ingredients, and cuisines to keep your meals exciting and satisfying.

The Future of Plant-Based Protein

As the world shifts toward more sustainable and health-conscious eating habits, the future of plant-based proteins looks bright. Food scientists are continually innovating to create delicious, realistic meat alternatives that appeal to even the most dedicated carnivores.

Plant-based protein options are becoming more accessible in restaurants, grocery stores, and fast-food chains, making it easier than ever to enjoy a protein-rich, plant-based diet.

By incorporating a variety of plant-based proteins into your meals, you can enjoy a sustainable, flavorful, and nutritious way of eating that benefits both your health and the planet. So, why not explore the vibrant world of plant-based proteins and discover the delicious possibilities they offer? Your taste buds and the environment will thank you.

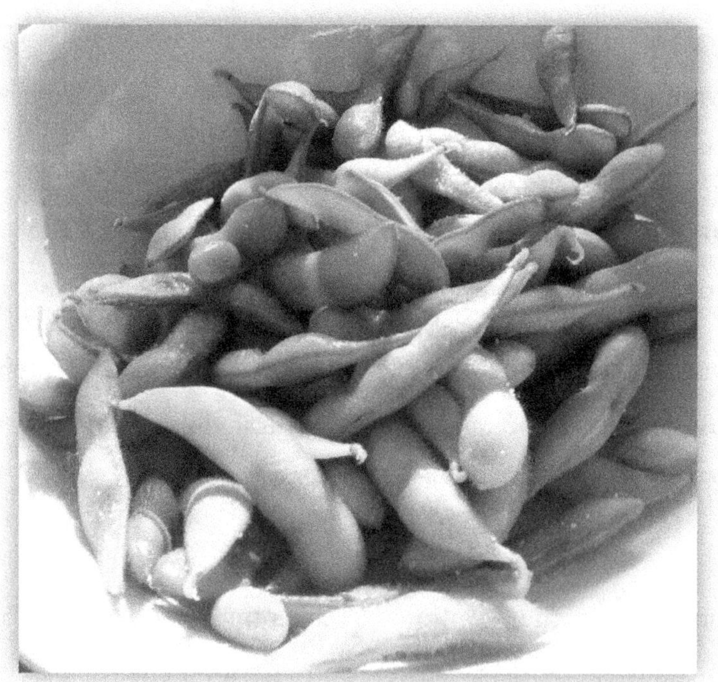

CHAPTER 8

Sip to Slim: Smart Beverage Choices

When it comes to maintaining a healthy lifestyle and achieving your weight loss goals, what you drink is just as important as what you eat. In this chapter, we'll explore the world of beverages and discover how to make smart choices that support your journey towards a slimmer, healthier you.

The Hidden Calories in Beverages

One common mistake many people make is underestimating the number of calories in their drinks. It's easy to focus solely on the calories in solid foods while overlooking the liquid calories that can quickly add up. Let's break down some popular beverages and their calorie content:

Soda: A regular 12-ounce can of soda can contain around 140 calories, mainly from added sugars. Opting for diet soda may save you calories but isn't necessarily a healthier choice due to artificial sweeteners.

Fruit Juice: While fruit juices may seem healthy, they can be calorie-dense. A small 8-ounce glass of orange juice contains approximately 120 calories, and many fruit juices have added sugars.

Energy Drinks: These beverages can pack a calorie punch, with some brands containing over 200 calories per 16-ounce serving, along with caffeine and added sugars.

Alcohol: Beer, wine, and cocktails can vary widely in calorie content. A light beer may have around 100 calories, while a single mixed drink can range from 100 to 300 calories or more.

Coffee Shop Specials: Those enticing coffee shop drinks can be laden with calories. A grande (16-ounce) café mocha with whipped cream can have over 400 calories.

The Power of Hydration

Water is the ultimate hydrator, and it plays a crucial role in weight management. Here's how staying hydrated can aid your weight loss efforts

Appetite Control: Drinking water before meals can help control your appetite, leading to reduced calorie intake during the meal.

Metabolism Boost: Staying properly hydrated supports your metabolism, helping your body burn calories more efficiently.

Thermogenesis: Cold water, in particular, can increase thermogenesis, the process by which your body burns calories to generate heat.

Toxin Elimination: Water helps flush toxins from your body, which can aid in overall health and weight management.

Healthy Beverage Choices

Now that we've covered the pitfalls, let's discuss how to make smart beverage choices that align with your weight loss goals:

Water: Make water your primary beverage of choice. It's calorie-free, refreshing, and essential for overall health.

If plain water isn't appealing, add a slice of lemon, lime, or cucumber for flavor.

Herbal Teas: Herbal teas like green tea, chamomile, and peppermint are excellent options. They're naturally caffeine-free and can be enjoyed hot or cold.

Infused Water: Create your own infused water by adding fresh fruits, herbs, or cucumber slices to a pitcher of water. This adds a subtle flavor without extra calories.

Sparkling Water: If you crave the fizz of soda, opt for sparkling water with a splash of citrus for flavor

Low-Fat Milk or Dairy Alternatives: For calcium and protein, choose low-fat or unsweetened plant-based milk like almond or soy.

Limit Alcohol: If you drink alcohol, do so in moderation. Choose lighter options like wine or light beer, and be mindful of portion sizes.

Read Labels: Check the nutrition labels on beverages, especially for added sugars and artificial additives. Avoid high-calorie, sugary drinks.

Portion Control Matters

In addition to making healthy beverage choices, portion control is key. Be mindful of the size of your drink servings, especially when ordering at restaurants or coffee shops. Opt for the smallest size available, share a large drink with a friend, or ask for a to-go cup to save half for later.

Stay Consistent

Consistency is crucial when it comes to beverages. Making smart choices most of the time can significantly impact your overall calorie intake. Keep a water bottle with you during the day to stay hydrated and reduce the temptation to reach for sugary drinks.

By paying attention to what you drink and making thoughtful choices, you can support your weight loss journey and overall well-being. Remember that every sip counts, so choose wisely, stay hydrated, and sip your way to a slimmer, healthier you.

CHAPTER 9

Mindful Eating: The Art of Eating for Health

In our fast-paced world, where we're constantly bombarded with distractions, it's easy to overlook one of life's most fundamental activities: eating.

Many of us rush through meals, eat in front of screens, or grab quick bites on the go. This often leads to mindless eating, where we're disconnected from the experience of nourishing our bodies. In this chapter, we'll explore the concept of mindful eating and how it can transform your relationship with food, promote weight loss, and enhance your overall well-being.

Understanding Mindful Eating

Mindful eating is a practice rooted in mindfulness, an ancient Buddhist concept that involves paying full attention to the present moment without judgment. When applied to eating, it means being fully present and aware of the entire eating experience, from selecting your food to savoring each bite.

Here's what mindful eating entails

Sensory Awareness: Engaging all your senses while eating. This means noticing the colors, textures, smells, and flavors of your food.

Paying Attention: Focusing solely on eating during meals, rather than multitasking or eating in front of the TV or computer.

Listening to Your Body: Tuning in to your body's hunger and fullness cues. This helps you eat when you're genuinely hungry and stop when you're satisfied, preventing overeating.

Chewing Thoroughly: Taking the time to chew your food slowly and savor each bite. This aids digestion and allows you to enjoy your food fully.

Mindful Food Choices: Making conscious choices about what you eat, considering both nutritional value and personal preferences.

The Benefits of Mindful Eating

Practicing mindful eating can have a profound impact on your health and weight loss journey:

Weight Management: Mindful eating encourages a healthier relationship with food, reducing impulsive eating and emotional eating, both of which can lead to weight gain.

Improved Digestion: Chewing food thoroughly aids digestion and nutrient absorption, reducing digestive discomfort.

Enhanced Enjoyment: By savoring each bite, you can find greater pleasure in your food and are less likely to seek satisfaction in unhealthy treats

Better Food Choices: Mindful eaters tend to make healthier food choices, as they are more attuned to their body's needs and preferences.

Stress Reduction: Practicing mindfulness during meals can reduce stress and promote relaxation.

How to Practice Mindful Eating

Start Small: Begin by dedicating just one meal or snack each day to mindful eating. Gradually increase the frequency as it becomes a habit.

Eliminate Distractions: Turn off screens, put away books or work, and create a quiet, focused eating environment.

Engage Your Senses: As you eat, notice the colors, textures, smells, and flavors of your food. Try to identify all the ingredients in a dish.

Chew Slowly: Take your time to chew each bite thoroughly. Put your utensils down between bites.

Listen to Your Body: Pause during your meal to check in with your hunger levels. Are you still hungry, or are you satisfied? Learn to recognize the signs of fullness.

Appreciate Your Food: Consider the effort and resources that went into producing your meal. Express gratitude for your nourishment.

Non-Judgmental Awareness: Be kind and non-judgmental toward yourself. If you notice your mind wandering, gently bring your focus back to your meal.

Mindful Food Choices: When selecting your meals, consider their nutritional value and how they make you feel. Choose foods that nourish your body and satisfy your taste buds.

Cultivating Mindful Eating Habits

Mindful eating is a skill that requires practice and patience. Over time, it can become a natural part of your daily routine, leading to a healthier relationship with food and supporting your weight loss and wellness goals.

By approaching each meal with mindfulness, you'll not only make more conscious food choices but also savor the joys of eating. It's a powerful tool in your journey toward a healthier, happier you. So slow down, savor your food, and embrace the art of mindful eating. Your body and mind will thank you.

CHAPTER 10

The Road Ahead: Sustainability and Long-Term Health

As you reflect on your progress so far, it's crucial to shift your focus towards long-term well-being and maintaining the positive changes you've made. In this final chapter, we'll explore the principles of sustainability and how they can ensure your continued success on the path to a healthier, happier you.

The Importance of Sustainability

Sustainability is about creating lasting habits and practices that contribute to your overall health and well-being. It's the opposite of quick-fix diets or short-term solutions.

Instead, it's a commitment to long-lasting change that supports not only your physical health but also your emotional and mental well-being.

Here's why sustainability matters

Preventing Weight Cycling: Sustainable habits help prevent weight cycling, the pattern of losing and regaining weight, which can be detrimental to your health.

Consistency Over Perfection: Sustainable habits allow for flexibility and balance in your life, so you're less likely to feel deprived or restricted.

Embracing Enjoyable Practices: Sustainable choices are those you can enjoy and maintain, making it more likely that you'll stick with them in the long run.

Keys to Long-Term Success

Set Realistic Goals: While it's essential to aim high, ensure your goals are realistic and achievable. Small, consistent steps are more sustainable than drastic changes.

Celebrate Milestones: Acknowledge and celebrate your successes along the way. Reward yourself for reaching milestones, but choose rewards that align with your health goals.

Stay Mindful: Continue practicing mindful eating and being aware of your body's hunger and fullness cues. This helps prevent overeating and emotional eating.

Regular Physical Activity: Incorporate physical activity into your daily routine. Find activities you enjoy, so staying active becomes a natural part of your life.

Diversify Your Diet: Keep your meals interesting by exploring new foods, recipes, and cuisines. Variety ensures you get a broad spectrum of nutrients.

Seek Support: Whether it's from friends, family, or a support group, having a network of people who share your health goals can be incredibly motivating and comforting.

Learn from Setbacks: Understand that setbacks are a natural part of any journey. Instead of being discouraged, use them as opportunities to learn and adjust your approach.

Balancing Health and Life

Sustainability is not about perfection; it's about balance. It's crucial to find equilibrium between your health goals and the other aspects of your life, such as work, family, and social activities. Here are some strategies:

Plan Ahead: Schedule time for meal preparation and exercise in your daily or weekly routine to ensure they don't get sidelined by other commitments

Communication: Talk to your friends and family about your health goals so they can provide support and understanding.

Flexibility: Be open to adjustments in your routine when necessary. Life is unpredictable, and sometimes you may need to adapt your plans.

Self-Compassion: Be kind to yourself. If you have an off day or make less-than-ideal choices, it's okay. Remember that each day is a new opportunity to make better choices.

The Continuation of Your Journey

Your journey to better health and sustainable weight management is not finite; it's a lifelong adventure. Along the way, you'll encounter new challenges and discoveries. Embrace them as opportunities to grow and refine your approach to health.

Remember that your health is an investment in your future self, and the choices you make today will impact your well-being for years to come. By focusing on sustainability, celebrating your achievements, and staying mindful of your body's needs, you're well-equipped to navigate the road ahead with confidence and vitality.

As you continue on this path, take a moment to appreciate how far you've come. You've gained valuable knowledge, developed healthier habits, and nurtured a more profound connection with your body. With sustainability as your compass, you're ready to embrace a future filled with health, vitality, and well-being. Here's to the journey ahead!

Conclusion

Your Journey to Vibrant Living

Congratulations on completing your journey through *Eat Well, Live Vibrantly.* You've embarked on a transformative adventure towards better health, increased vitality, and a more vibrant life. This guide has equipped you with valuable knowledge about the foods that nourish your body and support your weight loss goals. But it's not just about what you eat; it's about how you live.

A Holistic Approach to Health

Throughout this guide, you've learned that true well-being is not achieved through crash diets or extreme measures. It's a holistic approach that considers not only what you put on your plate but also how you nourish your mind and spirit. Here are some key takeaways:

Mindful Eating: The practice of mindful eating has empowered you to build a more profound connection with your body and its needs.

By listening to your hunger and fullness cues, you've established a healthier relationship with food.

Nutrient-Rich Foods: You've discovered the power of whole, nutrient-dense foods. These foods not only support your weight loss journey but also fortify your body against illness and disease.

Balance and Moderation: Sustainability is the cornerstone of lasting change. By finding balance in your life and practicing moderation, you've set yourself up for long-term success.

Physical Activity: Incorporating physical activity into your daily routine is a celebration of what your body can achieve. It's not just about burning calories; it's about embracing movement as a source of joy and vitality.

Embracing Variety: Your exploration of diverse cuisines and ingredients has made eating a more exciting and enjoyable experience. Variety ensures you receive a wide spectrum of nutrients.

The Power of Choice

As you move forward on your journey, remember that every meal is an opportunity to make choices that align with your health goals. It's about choosing nourishment over deprivation, self-care over neglect, and vitality over stagnation. Your choices are a reflection of your commitment to living vibrantly.

A Vibrant Future Await

Your journey towards vibrant living doesn't end here. It's an ongoing adventure, filled with new discoveries, challenges, and triumphs. Embrace each day as an opportunity to nurture your body and soul. Celebrate your successes, learn from your setbacks, and always be kind to yourself.

Surround yourself with a community of support, whether it's friends, family, or fellow health enthusiasts. Share your knowledge and experiences, and let your journey inspire others to embark on their path to vibrant living.

Remember that vibrant living is not a destination; it's a way of life. It's waking up each day with gratitude for the chance to nourish your body, mind, and spirit. It's savoring the flavors of whole foods, moving with intention, and nurturing your inner well-being.

As you step into the future, know that you have the tools, knowledge, and inner strength to overcome any obstacle and continue thriving. Your vibrant life is waiting for you to embrace it fully. So, go forth with confidence, purpose, and a heart filled with the joy of living vibrantly.

www.ingramcontent.com/pod-product-compliance
Lightning Source LLC
Chambersburg PA
CBHW080942260726
48661CB00010B/4043